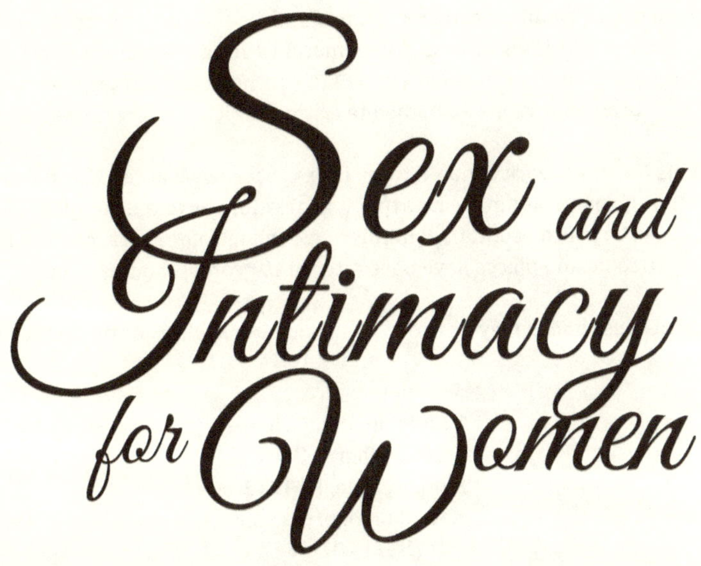

Sex and Intimacy for Women

The Secrets of Great Pleasure in and out of the Bed

Jenn Hodge, RN

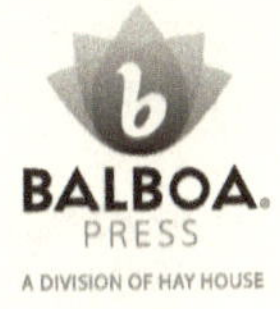

BALBOA.
PRESS

A DIVISION OF HAY HOUSE

Balboa Press books may be ordered through booksellers or by contacting:

Balboa Press
A Division of Hay House
1663 Liberty Drive
Bloomington, IN 47403
www.balboapress.com
1 (877) 407-4847

Print information available on the last page.

ISBN: 978-1-9822-0215-6 (sc)
ISBN: 978-1-9822-0216-3 (e)

Library of Congress Control Number: 2018904282

Balboa Press rev. date: 07/09/2018

The material in the book may include information by third parties. Third party materials comprise of opinions expressed by their owners. As such, the author of this book does not assume responsibility or liability for any third party material or opinions.

The publication of third party material does not constitute the author's guarantee of **any** information, products, services, or opinions contained within third party material. Use of third party material does not guarantee that your results will mirror our results. Publication of such third party material is simply a recommendation and expression of the author's own opinion of that material.

Whether because of the progression of the Internet, or the unforeseen changes in company policy and editorial submission guidelines, what is stated as fact at the time of this writing may become outdated or inapplicable later.

This book is copyright ©2017 by **Jenn Hodge RN & Edwardo Rosso** with all rights reserved. It is illegal to redistribute, copy, or create derivative works from this book whole or in parts. No parts of this report may be reproduced or retransmitted in any forms whatsoever without the written expressed and signed permission from the author.

Contents

Introduction

Thank you for taking the time to read and understand this fantastic guide— **"SEX & INTIMACY FOR WOMEN: The Secrets of Great Pleasure in & Out of the Bed."**

This Publication is intended for women to understand intimate relationships with their partner. Please note that men also have a role which will be discussed in our next book. Remember it takes two to tango!

Our Current Reality:

Studies show that there are four things that people want most in life. Financial freedom, better health, to look good and engaging in harmonious relationships. Today, we are going to focus on how to have a more harmonious, intimate relationship.

My intention for you is to have a better understanding of how relationships flow and work. Once you gain this understanding, you have no idea the power you can own for yourself.

Unfortunately, currently over 50% of marriages end in divorce. The other 50% who are still married, approximately a sad 20% are happy. I am part of the 50% who got divorced and am here to help you avoid the mistakes that I made and the heartache I endured.

I am blessed to have learned the secret of how relationships work and how to gain respect from your man in and out of the bedroom. Once I share these tips and tools with you he will have eyes for you and only you! Yes, I understand men like to look, that's human nature. He may glance from time to time but will never stray because of the knowledge and skill you now possess. If your marriage or relationship is on the rocks give this a try, you just may save your relationship by applying even a few strategies in this book!

Let's Get Started!

Types of Relationships

CONTRARY TO THE GENERAL belief that some relationships are good and some are bad or possibly even toxic, we are all seeking the relationships that serve us best. If we choose a different approach and better understand relationships, we may see them as a tool to better ourselves. Then we can make necessary changes that will allow us to become better communicators and perhaps improve our ability to respond to situations more effectively.

WHAT IS THE PURPOSE OF RELATIONSHIPS?

The purpose of all relationships is growth and evolution, which means every relationship serves a purpose. Even if you consider a relationship to be terrible and to have no value it will still occur to help you learn, grow and evolve. Please do not discount any relationship you experience. Always be ready to face the next one and be open to experience, learn and grow.

There are several types of relationships. The first category I would like to discuss is our relationship with the environment. In this relationship, we must obey to the laws of nature, even if we don't feel like it. The law of nature does not care who you are, and if you choose to jump off a high building, you will die because you did not obey to the law of gravity.

If you decide not to eat nature will kill you. If you choose not to sleep the law of nature will kill you, so inevitably you don't have much of a choice. Again, it is in your best interest to obey to the laws of nature as much as possible. Some more examples include -eating natural food that is fresh and pure to fuel your body. Protecting yourself from cold and heat when needed, so your body does not become frostbitten or dehydrated and getting regular exercise for if you choose to stay sedentary, your muscles will atrophy.

There are also relationships with others such as friends, coworkers and family members. Wouldn't it be nice to understand relationships better so you can communicate with your children, parents, and friends more effectively? In relationships with others, it is important that we respect each other. If we can be open to listening to other people's experiences and opinions, we can then learn from and collaborate with them. Why wouldn't you want to learn from another's experiences?

Their knowledge can help you possibly avoid the same mistakes or get to your desired goal faster because of their lessons. As you can see relationships are incredibly complex.

They require understanding so you don't fall into the trap of just abandoning them and missing out on the opportunity of your learning, growth, and evolution. "Relationships are everything and everything is a relationship so in life they are unavoidable."

INTIMATE RELATIONSHIPS AND THE DIFFERENCES BETWEEN MEN AND WOMEN

Also in this book we are focusing on another type of relationship, an intimate relationship between a man and a woman. The first point that is not well understood is that men and women are different both physiologically and psychologically.

A man has a penis and a scrotum, and a woman has a vagina and breasts. Although this may appear to be common sense, there is more to it than meets the eye.

A man has more muscle mass and strength than a woman. The areas of the body that feel the most pleasure are also different on a man than on a woman. To please each other, we need to be aware of where those areas are located. Unfortunately, we tend to fall short in teaching and sharing so that our partner can please us entirely.

We then spend a lot of time complaining that we did not receive the pleasure we expected or wanted. We then blame our partner when we truly have no one to blame but ourselves. I will share with you later in this publication exactly where the points on the body are for both men and women so you can both experience explosive pleasure like never before!

Men and woman are also different psychologically. Women tend to want more of a connection with their partner. They need to feel nurtured and desired. Men, because of their high testosterone level need sex and want to feel that they are adequately providing for their woman in and out of the bedroom.

Without this desire to procreate, our species would die out, so nature has made certain that will not happen.

It is the woman's job to make sure her man keeps coming back to her and only her, and it begins outside the bedroom. Then during sex she has a significant role. Before we explore that role, let's talk about the many benefits of sex.

Benefits of Sex

REGULAR SEX CANNOT BE underestimated as a factor for reducing stress, bolstering self-esteem and bonding that occurs between partners. The real point of this publication is the fact that a healthy sex life can provide for a longer, healthier, and most would agree, a more enjoyable life. Sex significantly relieves stress, emotionally and physically.

Sex and orgasm flood the body with good feeling chemicals called beta-endorphins which are great healers. These hormones can boost your immune system which spends its entire life fighting off bacteria, viruses, and diseases such as heart disease, high blood pressure, IBS, fibromyalgia, GERD and even cancer.

Disease occurs when the body becomes out of balance because stress has risen to an intolerable level. Why wouldn't you want to give your body every possibility to be healthy?

THE TOP ELEVEN HEALTH BENEFITS OF SEX

1. Improved Immunity and a Healthy Glow

People who have sex frequently (three times a week) have significantly higher levels of immunoglobulin A (IgA). Your IgA immune system is your body's first line of defense.

It's job is to fight off invading organisms at their entry points, reducing or even eliminating the need for activation of your body's immune system. It may explain why people who have sex frequently also take fewer sick days.

There's nothing sexy and inviting about sneezing, wheezing, or a red, runny nose. But getting hot and bothered can help you avoid coming down with a cold or flu bug. According to researchers at Wilkes University in Pennsylvania, these antibodies help combat diseases and keep the body safe from colds and flu. Save up your sick days and stay in bed for some healthy sex.

Sex helps you have and maintain a youthful, healthy glow. In a study conducted at the Royal Edinburgh Hospital in Scotland, a panel of judges viewed participants through a one-way mirror and guessed their ages.

Those who were enjoying lots of sex with a steady partner four times a week, were on average perceived to be seven to twelve years younger than their actual age. Regular sex promotes the release of hormones, including testosterone and estrogen, which can keep the body looking young and vital; estrogen has also been shown to promote soft skin and shiny hair. Why not add regular sex to your skin care regimen?

2. Heart Health

Sex counts as cardio! A romp in the hay can burn anywhere from 85 to 250 calories, depending on the length of the session. Obviously, a quickie will be less strenuous than an all-nighter. In fact, cardiologists consider sexual activity comparable to a modest workout on a treadmill, according to a study published in The American Journal of Cardiology.

3. Lower Blood Pressure

Sexual activity, specifically intercourse, is linked to lower blood pressure. Can you think of a better way to reduce your blood pressure?

4. Sex Is a Form of Exercise

Sex helps to boost your heart rate, burn calories and strengthen muscles, just like exercise. In fact, research recently revealed that sex burns about four calories a minute for men and three for women, making it, at times, a significant form of exercise. Sex can even help you to maintain your flexibility and balance.

5. Pain Relief

Sexual activity releases pain-reducing hormones and has been found to help reduce or block back and leg pain, as well as pain from menstrual cramps, arthritis, and headaches.

One study even found that sexual activity can lead to partial or complete relief of headaches in some migraine and cluster-headache patients. The surge of hormones released after an orgasm can help ease any annoying ache, whether it's a strained back or a horrible migraine.

A study conducted at the Headache Clinic at Southern Illinois University found that half of female migraine sufferers reported relief after climaxing. The endorphins that are released during an orgasm closely resemble morphine, and they relieve pain.

Have a migraine, but your man isn't around? Self-medicate by treating yourself with some solo sex. As long as you hit your peak, masturbating will have the same soothing effect.

6. May Help Reduce Risk of Prostate Cancer

Research has shown that men who ejaculate at least twenty-one times a month during sex or masturbation - have a lower risk of prostate cancer.

7. Improves Sleep

Don't go to bed angry. The stress on your body is not worth it. Your body requires six to eight hours of quality sleep. It is not healthy to lay awake stewing over an argument. It is okay to agree to disagree and then have makeup sex to release all of the stress. You will go to sleep relaxed and have the best night ever!

After sex, the relaxation-inducing hormone prolactin is released, which may help you to nod off more quickly.

Oxytocin, which is considered the love hormone, is released during orgasm and also promotes sleep.

It's downright dreamy how an orgasm can lull you to sleep. That's because the same endorphins that help you de-stress can also relax your mind and body, priming you for slumber, says Dr.Cindy M. Meston director of the Sexual Psychophysiology Laboratory at the University of Texas at Austin.

Plus, during orgasm the hormone prolactin is released. "Prolactin levels are naturally higher when we sleep, which suggests a strong relationship between the two," she says. But if you're wild in bed, please remember that; highly active sex can make you feel more energized than sleepy.

8. Stress Relief

Sex is significant to a relationship and stress relief of both parties. Sex triggers your body to release its natural feel-good chemicals, helping to ease stress and boost pleasure, calm and self-esteem. Research also shows that those who have sexual intercourse responded better when subjected to stressful situations like speaking in public.

If you are stressing over tomorrow's job interview, slip between the sheets. Research from the University of the West of Scotland reveals that people who had intercourse at least once over two weeks were better able to manage stressful situations such as public speaking, says study author and psychology professor Dr. Stuart Brody.

That's because endorphins and oxytocin are released during sex, and these feel-good hormones activate pleasure centers in the brain that create feelings of intimacy and relaxation and help stave off anxiety and depression, says WH advisor Dr. Laura Berman, an assistant clinical professor of ob-gyn and psychiatry at the Feinberg School of Medicine at Northwestern University.

You don't have to climax to net the effects, but you'll get the biggest surge of soothing hormones if you have an orgasm. Just one more reason to understand and practice the skills you are about to learn. The probability and the number of orgasms a woman will experience can significantly increase by applying the techniques in this book.

9. Boost Your Libido

The more often you have sex, the more likely you are to want to keep doing it. There's both a mental and physical connection, particularly for women. More frequent sex helps to increase vaginal lubrication, blood flow and elasticity, which in turn makes sexual activity more enjoyable.

10. Improved Bladder Control in Women and a Decrease in PMS

Intercourse helps to strengthen your pelvic floor muscles which contract during orgasm. It can help women to improve their bladder control and avoid incontinence. "When a woman orgasms, her uterus contracts and, in the process, rid the body of cramp-causing compounds.

The increased number of uterine contractions can also help expel blood and tissue more quickly, contributing to ending your period faster. Who wouldn't want lighter, shorter periods with less cramping?!

Engaging in intercourse while menstruating has also been shown to help decrease the risk of endometriosis, a common condition in which uterine tissue grows outside of the uterus, causing pelvic pain and sex that hurts, according to researchers at Yale University School of Medicine.

Sex during your period may not sound too appealing, but don't stress over making a mess. Just lay down a dark-colored towel and stick to missionary. When you're lying down, your flow tends to be lighter, says WH advisor Dr. Michelle Callahan.

11. Increase Intimacy and Improve your Relationship

Sex and orgasm result in increased levels of the hormone oxytocin, the "love" hormone, that helps you feel bonded to your partner and better experience empathic connections.

"Having sex regularly can do more than make you feel closer to your partner it can contribute to you becoming physically healthier," says Dr. Hilda Hutchinson, a clinical professor of obstetrics and gynecology at Columbia University.

What Gets in the Way of Frequent Sex?

I UNDERSTAND SOMETIMES YOU ARE tired and also may have a headache but if this becomes the norm, there is a problem. You deny yourself, not just your partner. If for some reason you are not in the mood and on occasion that's ok, just be aware your man is always in the mood. Sometimes you may have to please your partner just by masturbating him for 15 minutes or so until he ejaculates. Trust me, he will be calmer and more pleasant, so it is well worth your effort.

There is another occurrence that appears to get in the way of couples having regular sex which is recommended to be practiced 2-4 times per week. When disagreements happen the last thing, you want to do is be intimate with your partner. Instead, you deny him and go to bed angry and may stay angry for days. It is hurting both of you and the relationship, especially the person who continues to hold onto that anger and frustration.

Emotions that don't feel good such as anger, fear, frustration, jealousy, etc. can cause the body to go down and the immune system to function at a less than optimal level. It opens you up to getting sick with a temporary illness or sometimes a chronic illness that may be with you for the rest of your life. The problem is that each one of us wants to be right and wants our way all of the time. Unfortunately, that's not how life works.

If you strive to be constantly right and it always has to be your way, or he always has to have his way there will be **MAJOR** constant conflict in your relationship.

This is the time where you ask yourself a crucial question, do I want to stay well or do I always have to be right? Take the time to listen to your partner and say something like, I can see your point can I think about this and get back to you tomorrow?

This will allow you both time to cool off and reflect on each other's perspective. In the meantime, have sex, you may even forget what the argument was all about! If one or both of you is having trouble with this concept, I suggest that some work may be needed to understand how life works and the difference between your physiology and psychology. Once you understand and apply the concepts in; The Manual 4 Life philosophy relationships will become much easier to navigate. This philosophy is available as a paperback and downloadable version on Amazon. For your convenience, I have included a link.

https://www.amazon.com/Manual-Life-Depth-Exploration-Consciousness-ebook/dp/B01L4SRN3I

We spend a ton of time as women trying to make ourselves more attractive to our man. We put on makeup and lipstick to have a more beautiful face. We wear heels with a mini-skirt so our legs look more toned and sexy. We wear a push-up bra, so our breasts look larger and are enhanced.

We spend so much time on this, but unfortunately our effort is wasted if we lack skill in the bedroom. I hate to break the news to you, but talent will win over a beautiful face and perfect body **EVERY SINGLE TIME, GUARANTEED**! If you improve your skills, your man will choose you over a model any day of the week. Don't believe me, try it for yourself and enjoy the benefits.

You must remember at one point seeing an ok looking woman with a gorgeous guy. Your first thought was how did she get him?! She has skill in the bedroom, plain and straightforward. Are you ready to learn and understand how to have and apply that skill with your man?

How to Have Amazing, Earth Shattering Sex

YOU MUST AGREE IF we are going to put in all of this effort we want to have great sex, not just standard, mediocre sex. The question is how? Guess what ladies it's all in your hands. Our role as women is so important because if we don't prepare him properly, he cannot perform well in the bedroom. Your skill is responsible for him:

1) Maintaining a reliable erection

2) Not experiencing premature ejaculation.

It is so important for you to understand that lack of a consistent erection in a man brings frustration and dissatisfaction to both partners. The man will not feel good enough because he can't stay hard and give you the orgasms you need. The woman feels equally not good enough because she feels he does not like her and is not excited for her; otherwise, he would be able to maintain his erection. This is fuel for a broken relationship.

The woman's role has the power to resolve this situation and bring harmony to both partners and the relationship.

I did not understand that I was the one in control of his erection and if I had this information may have contributed to saving my marriage. A man needs to stay hard and not ejaculate too quickly, or he cannot please you. Also, make sure your man knows he is pleasing you. Tell him you like it when he … and please let him know when you are having an orgasm! This will help him feel more like a man. If he does not feel like a man with you, the probability of him seeking for another woman outside of your relationship significantly increases. Now you can see how valuable this information can be.

I know a guy who loved his wife, but he never felt appreciated at home. He worked hard at his job and did not believe his wife noticed him at all. He knew his wife worked hard too, and he was not looking for a competition. She barely noticed when he cleaned up on the weekends or cooked dinner. He was beginning to feel a little worthless. To make matters worse, sex was becoming less and less frequent. She made excuses a lot to avoid sex, and when they did finally have sex, she barely seemed to enjoy it, never really expressing her enjoyment or pleasure during an orgasm.

One day his secretary noticed he was a little down and asked what was wrong. He told her what was happening without going into detail and she said his wife was making a huge mistake and that he was a great guy. She was not doing this in any way to benefit herself, she was just being nice.

As the weeks went on, he began confiding in his secretary more often, and they started to become closer. One late night at the office passion overtook them and they wound up having sex. For the first time in a very long time, he felt like a man. What was different about the encounter with his secretary and sex with his wife? His secretary screamed with pleasure and voiced loudly when she orgasmed, plus, she asked him for more!

Now, who do you think the man will continue to go back to, the woman that screams or the woman who continues to act bored during sex? If you guessed the woman who screams, you would win! Now, which woman would you like to be? It's your choice ladies and if a man does not feel like he pleases you he will feel incapable as a man. Let's now understand how to keep that man of yours in your arms and not the secretaries.

HOW TO ENGAGE IN AMAZING SEX

To begin your sexual encounter, it is important to relax each other before intercourse. Take some time to massage each other before beginning actual touching of more intimate parts of the body. I like to use regular massage to relax muscles and then practice a technique called **SSTT** (Super Slow Touch Technique).

You lightly stroke with one or two fingers very gently your partner's arms, legs, stomach, face, feet, etc. ... The woman should receive the massage first because once you start focusing on the man's genitals, you will be preparing him for intercourse. The massage itself can be 5 to10 minutes or however long you choose. Foreplay, where you are preparing the man to maintain his erection must be 15-20 minutes long and to get the results you desire, you must follow instructions carefully. Do not skimp and only have 10 minutes of foreplay because your sex will remain mediocre at best. Once you create a new habit, this will become simpler,, effortless and enjoyable!

THE SPOT

As I stated earlier men and woman feel pleasure in different parts of their genitals. A woman can experience extreme pleasure in her clitoris which is a small area above the vaginal opening with thousands of nerve endings. This tiny spot needs to be handled with care and responds best to very light strokes or touches. I have included a diagram below. I was not aware that some women don't know where their clitoris is and most men have no clue. So now you know by the diagram below and can share this information with your partner. The clitoris only has **ONE** function which is pleasure!

Anatomy of Human Vagina

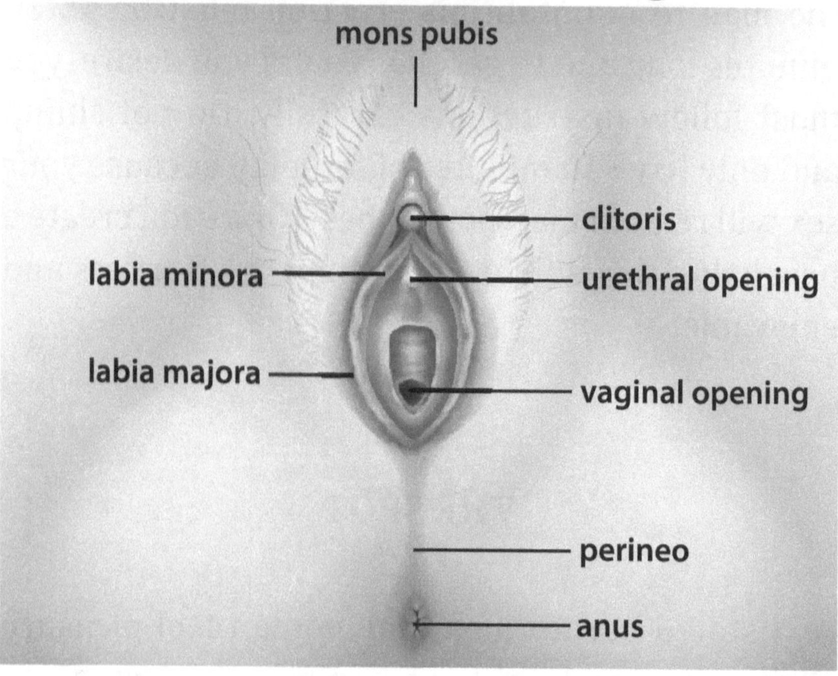

A man has one spot on the underside of his penis where he experiences all his pleasure. It is a thin cord that starts right below the glans of his penis and continues down approximately one inch.

If you do not focus on this spot when you are preparing your man either with your hands or mouth you are wasting your time. The head of the penis usually gets irritated when stimulated too much as well as the front side of the penis. Again, all your focus needs to be on the spot.

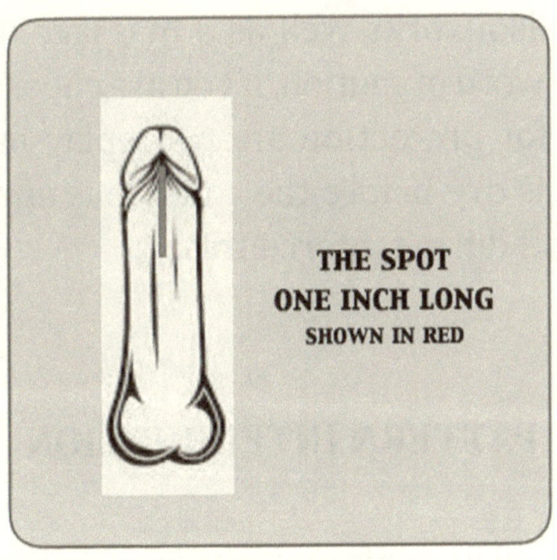

LUBRICATION

Lubrication is of utmost importance during foreplay and also during actual intercourse. I have found that good ole natural (preferably organic) olive oil makes the best lubricant. It is a natural anti-inflammatory which can help the vagina not get irritated from too much friction. The olive oil also helps increase the pleasure of the penis and clitoris during foreplay.

Also, during intercourse, if the vagina is too dry your man may have more difficulty maintaining his erection during initial penetration and that is a big problem for it can facilitate the loss of his erection. Feel free to be generous with the amount of olive oil you use. If you are concerned about staining the sheets, place a towel before getting started.

Olive oil also works well as a massage oil for the body. One word of caution, if you are choosing to use condoms for protection after foreplay make sure the penis is dry before the condom is applied or it may slip off during intercourse.

PATTERN INTERRUPTION

During foreplay, it is important to prepare your man for 15-20 minutes. It will keep him erect during intercourse and also help him to be able to last much longer so you can enjoy sex more and experience more orgasms. Practicing foreplay on your man for 15-20 minutes will also help avoid premature ejaculation by training his brain by interrupting the pattern often. It is where we as women need to become creative.

How many different ways can you think of to touch his penis either with your hands or mouth while **ALWAYS** focusing on the spot, as referenced above?

You can use a full stroke, and you can use your tongue, you can use your thumbs, you can use your palm, you can use a twisting motion, you can use your mouth (gently and lightly).

Again, make sure there is enough lubrication, and you are always hitting the spot.

Now for a lesson on pattern interruption. Each time you pick a pattern, full stroke, thumbs, tongue, etc ..., each move should be performed 20 times and then switch to a new pattern. You can go back to a pattern later, but if you stick to one for too long, he will ejaculate. Now, this is fine if that is your intention, but if it's not, you will be disappointed. You can also use pattern interruption during intercourse but in a slightly different way.

Switch things up a bit and try different positions. The same situation every single time can become extremely mundane so get creative and have a little fun. Pattern interruption is designed to help your man keep his erection for a very extended period of time. Let's explore a little more how to apply pattern interruption to benefit both of you.

As explained above, always focus on the spot (see above) on the penis. While you are using your same pattern with hands and also mouth for 20 times each, you must also maintain the same speed and same pressure while you are applying the same movement.

You will be guaranteed to reach more orgasms because you are retraining his brain and penis to not orgasm prematurely. Some of our students have experienced 15-20 orgasms per session on a regular basis by applying the techniques in this publication.

Remember, a man feels like a man not by the size of his penis but by the amount of orgasms he can produce for his woman. Because the above topic is of utmost importance, I would like to be confident you understand some key points. Sequencing is not only important in sex, but in everyday life.

Think about when you drive your car to work. You open the door, make sure you have the key, get in the car, close the door and finally start the engine and drive the vehicle. If any of these steps are forgotten, you will not get to work.

I know what you're thinking, that's ok I don't like my job anyway. But in all seriousness to accomplish anything in life, you need to follow a sequence and this includes sex. Now, let's understand the seqencing during sex by recapping the highlights below.

1. Massage and relax each other- The woman receives first (by her request) He will be happy to massage you because he knows he will be getting his reward later (sex).
2. Massage him with SSTT- (that's the super soft and slow strokes with one or two fingers) first

anywhere you desire and then focus only on his genitals. This will majorly relax him while turning him on at the same time.

3. 20-minute foreplay to build a firm erection and prevent premature ejaculation- Remember to use olive oil for lubrication and also interrupt the pattern after 20 times with one pattern, then switch to a new pattern.

4. Lubricate your vagina with olive oil- it is now time to begin intercourse. Choose any position you like, but whatever position you choose, I recommend starting slow.

5. Take breaks during sex but remember to continue stroking his penis while focusing on the spot- You can use SSTT on his penis at this time too. It will help his endurance escalate even more.

6. When you are complete, ask him for one more orgasm and let him know you are ready to hear his orgasm-Let him know if he is allowed to come inside you or if you will complete his orgasm with your hand or mouth. Do not let him do this himself! It will significantly decrease the pleasure he receives, and he will possibly stray if not satisfied.

7. This last step is essential- Spend 5-10 minutes holding each other and let him know how much

you enjoyed the amazing sex. You can perform SSTT on each other for a few minutes as well.

BREATH

Breath is life, and without it, we die. Breathing correctly during sex can help your sessions last longer so make sure you are inhaling and exhaling fully. Do not hold your breath during sex and especially not during orgasm. Also during foreplay, if you pay attention to your partners breathing you will know if he's getting too close to orgasm so make sure you are paying attention and remember to practice pattern interruption.

Also for the gentlemen, you can also know when your woman is climaxing by her breathing so you can help her reach her full orgasm by slightly speeding up.

VARIETY IS THE SPICE OF LIFE

One of the aspects of sex and intimacy is variety. Most couples when interviewed after being married or in a relationship for 2-3 years only practice one position during intercourse. Are you in this category?! People need variety in all aspects of life. Would you want to continue going to the same restaurant every single time you went out to dinner? Here are some suggestions but please feel free to be creative. (See pics below)

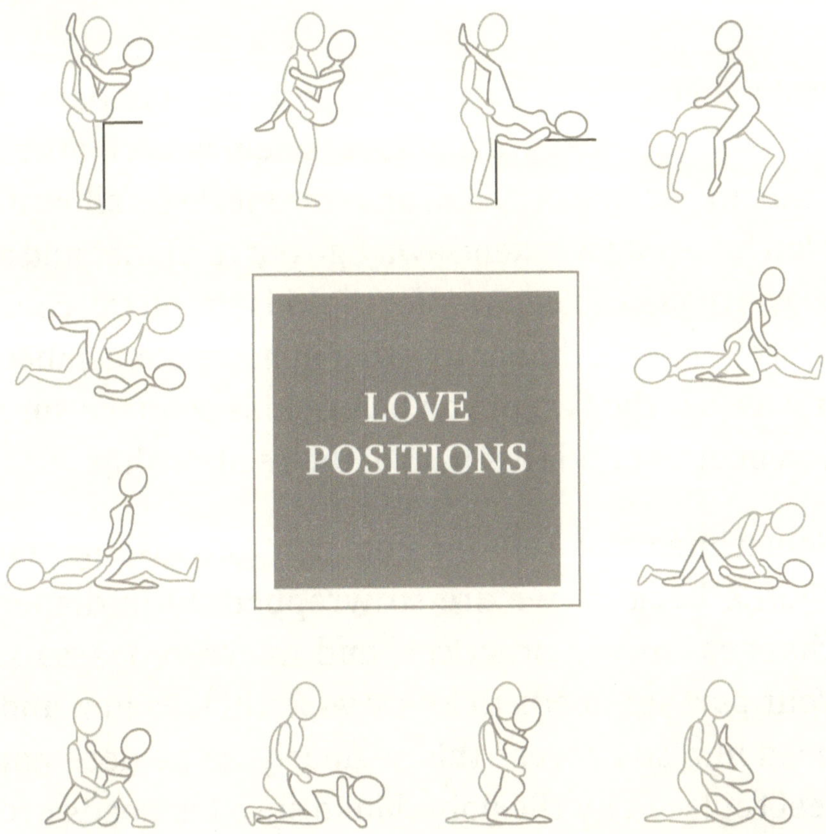

Variety can also include having sex in a different location, the living room floor in front of the fireplace for example or the gazebo out by the pool if the area is secluded enough. Also, if you always have sex in the morning, mix it up a little and have sex before bed or maybe in the afternoon before the kids come home from school. Again, here is your chance to become creative.

MAKE TIME FOR EACH OTHER

Make a chance to have fun together. A big part of life is about pleasure and love, so enjoy each other. Life can become very dull and routine if you allow it. Plan for a long weekend away, go out to dinner and a movie or plan a sleepover for the kids so you can cook a nice romantic dinner together at home. Remember, it was just the two of you before kids so make sure you bear in mind that part of the relationship.

Sometimes the relationship can get lost in the shuffle because we are so wrapped up in diaper changes, soccer practices, and dance rehearsals. Your partner needs to know you still love him and need him so express this regularly, so he does not feel replaced by the baby. Make sure his needs are still met emotionally and sexually. Yes, I know you are tired but trust me if he is happy he will be a lot more willing to run to the grocery store, take the 4 am feeding or cook you a nice dinner.

PLEASURE OUTSIDE THE BEDROOM

Now, let's apply what we learned in bed outside the bed. If you understand and acknowledge and apply this information to your psychology, it will help your life become richer outside the bedroom. Then you will indeed be experiencing life to the fullest. What do I mean by this?

I also want you to be able to experience extreme pleasure in your emotions. What makes you feel good in your emotions? Happiness, joy, peace, feelings of accomplishment, etc. It can be obtained by complimenting your spouse or significant other on a regular basis. What makes a man feel like a man is when he can please you and make you orgasm in bed. But if he does not please you outside the bed he also is not happy.

So how can we as women make sure our man knows we are pleased? Here is an example- you go on vacation and you know your partner saved money and worked overtime to bring you on a fantastic trip to the beach. He also made reservations at a few fancy restaurants and went out of his way to make you feel special.

REMEMBER TO BE THANKFUL

Please remember to thank him for his efforts and let him know how much you enjoyed the trip and dinners. You both will feel amazing, and he will want to do more for you. Another example- he surprises you on vacation with a shopping spree, and you feel like a queen for a day.

Let him know how special this made you feel. Now your man is complete for he can please you not only in the bedroom but outside as well. Do you think he will stray anywhere at this point? The answer is no. He's yours for life and the more you practice these tools, the more you will receive in and out of bed. Appreciation is a potent tool for everyone to apply. For more on recognition and step by step instructions on how to appreciate fully please read the chapter on appreciation in The Manual 4 Life philosophy. Available at:

https://www.amazon.com/Manual-Life-Depth-Exploration-Consciousness-ebook/dp/B01L4SRN3I

Conclusion

Men and women have various roles in the bedroom. Your job is to get him hard by practicing the skills learned above during 20-minute foreplay. These skills will help him not only obtain an erection but also to keep it during intercourse for a very long time so you can orgasm. His role is to perform in bed so he can please you. Without your skill, he is not able to perform well.

So again, it is nice to look and smell pretty, but the woman with skill will win the man **EVERY** time hands down! Also, please remember to tell your man you love him. Although he tries to be macho all the time, he still needs to know that he is appreciated and loved.

Now you can see how valuable this information is. If you would rather continue what you are doing, you have no one to blame but yourself if your sex life is boring and mediocre!

Now you have a bunch of new tools to spark up your relationship and keep it happy and healthy. Use the skills you have learned on a regular basis, and I promise you outstanding results.

You also have new tools to use outside the bedroom to experience a richer, fuller, happier life. I am so excited for you to begin your new journey with your partner and experience the most incredible pleasure you have ever had. May you use all you have learned here in good health! And don't worry, your man also has a role to please you in and out of the bedroom so he is not off the hook. This will be covered in book two in this series.

Namaste.

Bibliography

ABC/AFP, Sex before public speaking calms nerves, ABC Science

Chideya, Farai, Helpful Tips for the Bedroom, NPR

Robert, Teri, Orgasm, Migraines, and Headaches, Health Central

Sieczkowski, Cavin. Regular Sex Can Make You Look 7 Years Younger, Scientist Says, Huff Post

Steidly,Brandon, Sex leads to a longer life, https://sites.psu.edu/siowfa15/

Wira Dineen, Cari, The Hidden Health Benefits of Sex, Women's Health